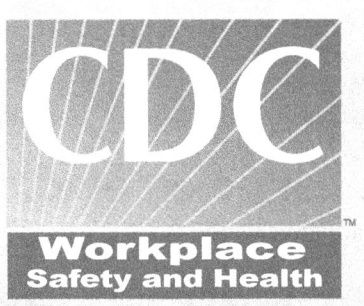

I0426025

Report on an Investigation of Buttermilk Flavoring Exposures and Respiratory Health at a Bakery Mix Production Facility

Gregory A. Day, PhD

Kristin J. Cummings, MD, MPH

Greg J. Kullman, PhD, CIH

Health Hazard Evaluation Report
HETA 2008-0230-3096
General Mills
Los Angeles, CA
November 2009

DEPARTMENT OF HEALTH AND HUMAN SERVICES
Centers for Disease Control and Prevention

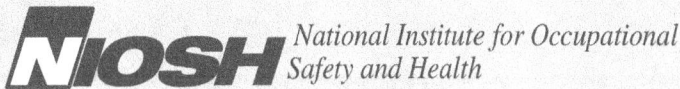 National Institute for Occupational Safety and Health

The employer shall post a copy of this report for a period of 30 calendar days at or near the workplace(s) of affected employees. The employer shall take steps to insure that the posted determinations are not altered, defaced, or covered by other material during such period. [37 FR 23640, November 7, 1972, as amended at 45 FR 2653, January 14, 1980].

CONTENTS

ABBREVIATIONS

ATS	American Thoracic Society
CA	California
CalOSHA	California Division of Occupational Safety and Health
CDC	Centers for Disease Control and Prevention
CI	confidence interval
DRDS	Division of Respiratory Disease Studies
ECRHS	European Community Respiratory Health Survey
°F	degrees Fahrenheit
FEV_1	forced expiratory volume in the first second of exhalation
FVC	forced vital capacity
HEPA	high-efficiency particulate aerosol
HHE	health hazard evaluation
IBT	International Brotherhood of Teamsters
L	liters
L/min	liters per minute
MDC	minimum detectable concentration
mg/m^3	milligrams per cubic meter of air
MQC	minimum quantifiable concentration
MSDS	material safety data sheet
NHANES III	Third National Health and Nutrition Examination Survey
NMAM	NIOSH Manual of Analytical Methods
NIOSH	National Institute for Occupational Safety and Health
OSHA	Occupational Safety and Health Administration
ppm	parts per million
ppb	parts per billion
PEL	permissible exposure limit
pDR	personal dataRAM
PID	photo-ionization detector
PNOR	particulates not otherwise regulated
PPE	personal protective equipment
PR	prevalence ratio
QRO	Quality and Regulatory Operation
RDHETAP	Respiratory Disease Hazard Evaluation and Technical Assistance Program
REL	recommended exposure limit
SAPP	sodium acid pyrophosphate
TWA	time-weighted average
VOC	volatile organic compound

HIGHLIGHTS OF THE NIOSH HEALTH HAZARD EVALUATION

NIOSH received a confidential request to conduct a health hazard evaluation (HHE) at the General Mills bakery mix production facility in Los Angeles, CA. Requesters were concerned about exposure to respiratory health hazards including flavorings containing diacetyl.

What NIOSH Did:

- Toured the facility.
- Interviewed plant management and company safety officials.
- Reviewed historical production records and material safety data sheets.
- Measured air concentrations of flavoring chemicals and respirable dust in various work areas.
- Measured exhaust ventilation system performance in the ingredients lab.
- Reviewed company logs of illness and injury.
- Interviewed 24 (59%) workers about their health and job histories, including 19 (70%) current production workers.
- Assessed 23 workers' lung function using spirometry, including 18 (67%) current production workers.

What NIOSH Found:

- A liquid buttermilk flavoring containing 15-20% diacetyl was used at the facility until mid-2008, when a re-formulated flavoring was introduced.
- The re-formulated buttermilk flavoring contains 2,3-pentanedione as the major substitute for diacetyl.
- Powered buttermilk flavorings containing 1% or less diacetyl are used at the facility.
- Diacetyl could be detected in the air in some work areas in the facility, but the concentrations were too low to measure using fully validated sampling and analytical methods.
- 2,3-pentanedione could be detected in the air in some work areas in the facility, and the concentration could be measured in one area of the production room where workers filled bags with dry bakery mix.
- Respirable dust concentrations throughout the facility were less than the permissible limit for particulates not otherwise regulated, but flavoring-containing dusts are not regulated and may be harmful.
- There were no cases of lung disease reported on company

logs of illness and injury.

- Some participants reported cough or nose, eye, or skin symptoms that improved away from work, indicating a work-related pattern.

- Ten (42%) participants reported asthma-like symptoms; 2 reported these symptoms improved away from work, indicating a work-related pattern.

- 22 lung function tests were interpretable: 18 (82%) were normal, 4 (18%) had a restrictive pattern, and none had an obstructive pattern.

- Participants had higher than expected rates of shortness of breath, ever receiving a physician's diagnosis of asthma, and restrictive pattern on spirometry, compared to U.S. adults.

What General Mills Managers Can Do:

- Avoid use of diacetyl-containing flavorings when possible.

- Until more is known about 2,3-pentanedione and similar alpha-diketone compounds, do not assume these compounds are safe.

- Communicate with workers about the health hazards of flavorings and the importance of limiting exposure to flavorings.

- Continue to require the use of half-face respirators with organic vapor cartridges during preparation of liquid flavorings in the ingredient room.

- Instruct workers to use N-95 filtering-facepiece or half-face respirators with particulate filters when performing tasks that generate dust.

- Use vacuum cleaners equipped with high-efficiency particulate aerosol (HEPA) filters as much as possible to clean residual powders from equipment.

- Encourage workers to report new, persistent, or worsening symptoms to their personal physician and to a designated individual at the workplace.

- Consider the use of serial spirometry to detect declines in lung function that may be due to flavorings.

In the past, some General Mills workers used a liquid buttermilk flavoring containing 15-20% diacetyl under conditions that may have resulted in exposure. Buttermilk flavorings currently used at the plant contain diacetyl substitutes and/or lower levels of diacetyl. None of the workers tested with spirometry had fixed airways obstruction seen in flavoring-related bronchiolitis obliterans. Because the toxicology of diacetyl substitutes is unknown and even low levels of diacetyl are potentially hazardous, workers' exposure to buttermilk flavorings should be limited through a combination of engineering controls, work practices, and respiratory protection.

What General Mills Workers Can Do:

- Follow work practices designed to limit exposure to flavorings, such as pouring liquid flavorings within the local exhaust ventilation hood.

- Wear appropriate respiratory protection as directed by management.

- Report new, persistent, or worsening symptoms to your personal physician and to a designated individual at the workplace.

NIOSH investigators conducted medical and industrial hygiene evaluations at the General Mills bakery mix production facility in Los Angeles, CA. A buttermilk flavoring containing 15-20% diacetyl was used at the facility in the past. Many currently used flavorings contain alpha-diketone substitute compounds, primarily 2,3-pentanedione, and/or lower concentrations of diacetyl. None of the workers tested with spirometry had fixed airways obstruction as seen in flavoring-related bronchiolitis obliterans. Participants had higher than expected rates of shortness of breath, physician-diagnosed asthma, and a restrictive pattern on spirometry, compared to U.S. adults. Some participants reported symptoms with a work-related pattern. Management should continue to limit exposures to flavorings through a combination of engineering controls, work practices, and respiratory protection. Workers should report symptoms to their personal physician and to a designated individual at the workplace.

On July 8, 2008, the National Institute for Occupational Safety and Health (NIOSH) received a confidential Health Hazard Evaluation (HHE) request to perform an investigation of possible health hazards at the General Mills, Inc. bakery mix facility in Los Angeles, CA. The requestors described concerns about respiratory health, including bronchiolitis obliterans which is a rare irreversible lung disease found in some workers exposed to diacetyl in flavorings. They noted exposure to hazardous chemicals, including flavorings containing diacetyl. Prior to their request, the California Division of Occupational Safety and Health (CalOSHA) had visited the facility, performing a limited review under the Flavoring Industry Safety and Health Evaluation Program. NIOSH investigators were aware that a buttermilk flavoring containing 15-20% diacetyl was used at the facility in the past, which had been re-formulated and reported to contain less than 1 percent diacetyl. NIOSH investigators conducted telephone interviews with workers, union representatives, an inspector from CalOSHA familiar with the facility, and company management and safety officials.

In September-October 2008, NIOSH staff conducted a medical survey at the plant consisting of an interviewer-administered questionnaire and lung function testing with spirometry before and after bronchodilator administration; they also observed production processes, collected bulk samples of flavorings, and measured concentrations of airborne contaminants in all areas of the facility. In May 2009, NIOSH staff performed additional air sampling to quantitate levels of a diacetyl substitute, 2,3-pentanedione.

NIOSH staff conducted spirometry on 24 (59%) of the current employees, including 19 (70%) production workers. None of the workers tested with spirometry had fixed airways obstruction as seen in flavoring-related bronchiolitis obliterans. Participants had higher than expected rates of shortness of breath, physician-diagnosed asthma, and a restrictive pattern on spirometry, compared to U.S. adults. Some participants reported symptoms with a work-related pattern.

Analytical results of headspace bulk samples of currently used liquid and powdered flavorings indicated that five of six contained the alpha-diketone substitute compound, 2,3-pentanedione; four contained diacetyl, three contained acetoin, and three contained other alpha-diketones. None of the applicable Material Safety Data Sheets for the evaluated bulk flavorings listed diacetyl or its alpha-diketone substitutes. Only one MSDS listed acetoin. Results of personal and area air samples indicated quantifiable concentrations of 2,3-pentanedione during handling of the re-formulated liquid buttermilk flavoring and during production of a bakery mix that contained the re-formulated flavoring. No diacetyl, acetoin, or other alpha-diketones were above minimum detection limits in workplace air for time-weighted samples.

The toxicology of diacetyl substitutes is only now being studied. Because 2,3-pentanedione, 2,3-hexanedione, and 2,3-heptanedione all share the same functional alpha-diketone group as diacetyl, these compounds may also share diacetyl's mechanism of toxicity. Until more is known about 2,3-pentanedione and other alpha-diketone compounds, they should not be assumed to be safe. A "safe" level of diacetyl has not been established, and even low levels of diacetyl are potentially hazardous. Management should continue to limit exposures to flavorings through a combination of engineering controls, work practices, and respiratory protection. Workers should report symptoms to their personal physician and to a designated individual at the workplace.

Keywords: Flavoring, diacetyl, 2,3-pentanedione, fixed obstruction, bronchiolitis obliterans, restrictive lung disease

On July 8, 2008, the National Institute for Occupational Safety and Health (NIOSH) received a confidential health hazard evaluation (HHE) request regarding the General Mills bakery mix production facility in Los Angeles, California. The requesters were concerned about the risks of asthma, bronchitis, bronchiolitis obliterans, eye irritation, and skin problems resulting from respiratory health hazards, including flavorings that contain diacetyl.

Diacetyl, a volatile diketone found in butter flavoring, was first recognized as a workplace health hazard at a microwave popcorn production plant [CDC 2002; Kreiss et al. 2002; Parmet, von Essen 2002]. Bronchiolitis obliterans, an irreversible obstructive lung disease, has since been detected throughout the microwave popcorn industry [Kanwal et al. 2006] and in flavoring and diacetyl manufacturing workers [CDC 2007; van Rooy 2007; NIOSH 2008]. As a safe level of diacetyl is currently unknown, protecting workers from flavorings-related lung disease requires limiting exposure through substitution, engineering controls, work practices, and personal protective equipment (PPE), along with medical surveillance using spirometry [NIOSH 2004; Kreiss 2007]. Chemicals used as diacetyl substitutes have poorly described toxicology and cannot be assumed to be safe. Therefore, limiting workers' exposure to diacetyl substitutes also is prudent.

Work-related asthma is well-recognized among bakery workers. Responsible allergens include wheat, rye, barley, buckwheat, and soy flours, as well as fungal enzymes such as alpha-amylase [Baur et al. 1998; Brisman 2002; Brant 2007]. Irritants likely also play a role [Baur et al. 1998; Brisman 2002]. Reduction of exposure through engineering controls such as local exhaust ventilation and work practices aimed at reducing dust generation are primary preventive steps [Brisman 2002].

Process Description

The General Mills facility in Los Angeles, California produces dry bakery mixes for commercial users. The facility has been in operation, under a variety of names, for more than 40 years. The operation, adjacent to a larger mill owned by another company, consists of a printweigh room, where dry ingredients are measured; a production room, where ingredients are combined and packaged; a warehouse area, where bulk ingredients, packaging and palletizing materials, and final products are stored, and an automatic palletizer is operated; a "Quality and Regulatory Operation" (QRO) laboratory, consisting of a kitchen where bakery products are prepared and tested for quality and an ingredient room where colorants and liquid flavorings are measured; and offices located in the other company's mill office building. The printweigh room, production room, and warehouse are located in one building and the laboratory and offices in another, connected by a bridge.

In the first step, some minor ingredients to be used during upcoming shifts are measured in the printweigh room and a few special ingredients in the laboratory. The printweigh worker measures out dry ingredients, such as baking soda, sodium acid pyrophosphate (SAPP), flavorings (including dry buttermilk flavoring containing up to 1% diacetyl), and enzymes, in 70 to 220 pound batches. Some ingredients are gravity fed, but most are transferred from storage containers using hand scoops. The printweigh room is equipped with local exhaust ventilation.

In a parallel step, a laboratory worker measures out colorants and liquid buttermilk flavorings in the ingredient room. Until mid-2008, the company used a liquid buttermilk flavoring containing 15-20% diacetyl for one product that was made every 4-6 weeks, but currently uses a re-formulated flavoring for this product. Over the last decade, the company has taken increasing steps to isolate the laboratory measuring tasks. Initially, colorants and liquid buttermilk flavoring were measured in the kitchen, with general exhaust only. Because the colorants tended to stain surfaces throughout the kitchen, the adjacent ingredient room was established. Over time, ventilation in the ingredient room has been upgraded from general exhaust to local exhaust to upgraded local exhaust with an additional ventilation hood, the most recent version of which was installed in 2007. An improved respiratory protection program for laboratory workers was introduced in 2007. Half-face negative-pressure respirators with organic vapor cartridges are used during handling of liquid flavorings.

Production workers (mixer operators) collect batches of dry powdered flavors from the printweigh room, transport them to the production room, and place them into downdraft ventilated hoppers along with flour, sugar, salt, and other solid ingredients. Mixer operators pour batches of liquid flavorings into a shortening tank by manually opening and closing a hinged lid, which occurs about three times per hour over the course of an eight-hour shift. Blending of all ingredients is an automated process that takes place in a closed bulk-mix delivery system; finished bake mixes are auger-fed into 50-pound bags, after which the bags are heat-sealed by packer operators and sent by conveyance to a palletizer.

The facility operates 24 hours per day in three shifts. At the time of our evaluation, the workforce consisted of 41 people: 27 production workers represented by the International Brotherhood of Teamsters (IBT) union, 3 laboratory workers, 4 supervisors, 1 local manager, 1 regional manager, and 5 office workers.

Prior to visiting the facility, NIOSH investigators conducted telephone interviews with company management and safety officials, union representatives, an inspector from the California Division of Occupational Safety and Health (CalOSHA) familiar with the facility, and several workers. In addition, we reviewed materials provided by the company, such as maps and material safety data sheets (MSDSs). To inform workers, we prepared a brief fact sheet about the HHE request and the planned NIOSH visit to the facility. This fact sheet was posted by the company at the facility and distributed to workers who provided a mailing address. We also called workers who provided a phone number.

Two physicians, two industrial hygienists, and three technicians from the NIOSH Division of Respiratory Disease Studies (DRDS) visited the facility from September 29 to October 2, 2008. Following a tour of the facility, we conducted medical and industrial hygiene surveys. Three industrial hygienists and a technician from NIOSH DRDS returned to the facility from May 26-27, 2009 to conduct additional industrial hygiene sampling.

Medical Survey

We invited all of the facility's employees to give written informed consent for a 15-minute interviewer-administered questionnaire and lung function testing. The questionnaire (Appendix A) included questions from the American Thoracic Society (ATS) adult respiratory questionnaire [Ferris 1978], the Third National Health and Nutrition Examination Survey (NHANES III) [CDC 1996], and the European Community Respiratory Health Survey (ECRHS) [Grassi et al. 2003]. Questions addressed respiratory and dermatological symptoms, asthma and other diagnoses, smoking history, work history and practices, and demographic information. We defined asthma-like symptoms as at least one of the following: wheezing or whistling in the chest in the past 12 months; being woken up with a feeling of tightness in the chest in the past 12 months; an attack of asthma in the past 12 months; or currently taking any medicine for asthma [Grassi et al. 2003]. Work-related asthma-like symptoms improved away from work.

The lung function testing consisted of spirometry with and without bronchodilator. Following ATS guidelines [Miller et al. 2005], a NIOSH technician administered spirometry tests using a dry rolling-seal spirometer interfaced to a personal computer. Bronchodilator consisted of four puffs of an inhaled beta-agonist administered to detect reversibility. A Spanish-speaking physician was available for participants who preferred to conduct the medical survey in Spanish.

We compared spirometry results to reference values generated from NHANES III data [Hankinson et al. 1999]. Each participant's largest forced vital capacity (FVC) and forced expiratory volume in 1 second (FEV_1) were selected for analysis. We classified participants as having obstruction if they had FEV_1/FVC ratio below the lower limit of normal with a normal FVC. We defined restriction as a normal FEV_1/FVC ratio with FVC below the lower limit of normal. We classified participants with both FEV_1/FVC ratio and FVC below the lower limit of normal as having mixed obstructive and restrictive abnormalities. FEV_1 determined severity, which ranged from borderline (FEV_1 above the lower limit of normal but below the predicted value) to very severe (percent predicted FEV_1 <35%). We defined reversibility as a 12% and 200 ml improvement in FEV_1 after bronchodilator administration [Pellegrino et al. 2005].

A report that explained each individual's spirometry results and provided recommendations for follow-up of abnormalities was mailed to each participant's home address within three weeks of testing. An interim letter summarizing the spirometry findings was sent to the company and requesters one month after our visit.

We calculated prevalence ratios (PRs) of respiratory symptoms, diagnoses, and spirometric classification from comparisons with the U.S. adult population prevalence reported in NHANES III [CDC 1996] using indirect standardization for race (white, black, or Mexican-American), sex, age (17-39 years or 40-69 years), and cigarette smoking status (ever or never). We explored associations between participants' work experiences and respiratory symptoms, diagnoses, and spirometric classification using contingency tables and the chi-square test for binary variables and Student's t-test for continuous variables.

Industrial Hygiene Surveys

On September 29, 2008, we observed the preparation of flavoring ingredients and production of bakery mixes, allowing us to obtain information on processes and controls. Key objectives in our sampling strategy were: 1) to collect bulk samples of flavorings, including the re-formulated liquid buttermilk flavoring; 2) to collect personal and area air samples during batch preparation of re-formulated liquid buttermilk flavoring; and 3) to collect personal and area air samples during production of the cake doughnut mix that contained the re-formulated liquid buttermilk flavoring.

On September 30 through October 2, 2008, we collected bulk samples of powdered and liquid ingredients, including the re-formulated liquid buttermilk flavoring, and a bulk sample of the cake doughnut mix that contained the re-formulated liquid buttermilk flavoring. We also measured contaminants generated during batch preparation of the re-formulated buttermilk flavoring and during production of the cake doughnut mix that contained the flavoring. Full-and partial-shift area air samples were collected for ketones (diacetyl and acetoin), aldehydes (acetaldehyde, benzaldehyde, and valeraldehyde), respirable dust, and volatile organic compounds (VOCs). Personal samples were also collected for the ketones, aldehydes, and respirable dust. Photo-ionization detectors (PIDs) were used to quantify real-time VOCs in air (RAE Systems Inc., Sunnyvale, CA). Real-time respirable dust measurements were made using PersonalDataRAM® monitors, model pDR-1000AN (Thermo Electron Corp., Franklin, MA). Samples were collected at different locations in the facility, including the QRO laboratory (ingredients room and kitchen), printweigh room, production room (mixing and packing areas), warehouse (palletizing area), and front offices. Additionally, we used smoke tubes to visualize air currents and evaluated ventilation systems by taking airflow measurements. Details on industrial hygiene sampling methods used during this survey are provided in Table 1.

On May 25 and 26, 2009, we used findings from the first industrial hygiene survey to perform another survey at the facility. Again, we measured contaminants generated during batch preparation of the re-formulated buttermilk flavoring and during production of the cake doughnut mix that contained the flavoring. We collected personal samples for ketones (diacetyl, acetoin, 2,3-pentanedione, 2,3-hexanedione, and 2,3-heptanedione) and area air samples for ketones and VOCs. PIDs were used to quantify real-time VOCs in air. All samples were collected at similar locations as those sampled in the first survey. Details on industrial hygiene sampling methods used during this second survey are provided in Table 2.

Medical Survey

A total of 24 (59%) of the facility's employees participated in the medical survey, including 19 (70%) production workers. Of employees who commonly handle flavorings, all 3 current laboratory workers, 2 of 3 current printweigh workers, and 3 of 5 current mixers participated.

The mean age of participants was 49 (range: 27-72) years and most (96%) were male. Fifteen participants (63%) identified their ethnicity as Hispanic. Thirteen participants (54%) identified their race as white, 5 (21%) as black, 1 (4%) as Asian, and 1 (4%) as Native Hawaiian or other Pacific Islander; 4 (17%) did not identify a race. Three (13%) participants were current smokers and 6 (25%) were former smokers. The median length of employment at the facility was 12 years (range: 1 – 35 years). The median length of employment in the current job was 6 years (range: 2 months – 25 years). The median number of hours worked in an average work week was 52 (range: 20-88 hours).

Table 3 details participants' experiences with buttermilk flavorings and flour during employment at the facility and in their current jobs. During employment, nearly all participants had worked with flour, two thirds had worked with powdered buttermilk flavorings, and half had worked with liquid buttermilk flavorings. In their current jobs, two thirds reported working with flour, half with powdered buttermilk flavorings, and one third with liquid buttermilk flavorings. While most who used flour in their current jobs did so daily, the use of buttermilk flavorings occurred on a less frequent basis (weekly to monthly). Two (8%) participants reported having used flavoring ingredients in jobs outside of the General Mills facility.

Twenty-two (92%) participants reported using a mask or respirator at the General Mills facility. The most common location for mask or respirator use was in the production room (n=19; 79%); other locations included the laboratory ingredient room (n=4; 17%), the printweigh room (n=3; 13%), and the warehouse (n=2; 8%). The most common task for mask or respirator use was "blowdowns," or cleaning with compressed air (n=12; 50%); other tasks included other types of cleaning (n=6; 25%) and when using flavorings (n=3; 13%). A total of 21 (88%) participants reported using compressed air for cleaning.

Table 4 presents the frequencies for reported chest (cough; shortness of breath; wheezing; chest tightness), nasal (stuffy, itchy, runny nose), eye (watery, itchy eyes), and skin (rash or other problem) symptoms. Some participants reported that their symptoms improved away from work, indicating a work-related pattern: 2 of 4 with usual cough, 1 of 4 with wheezing or whistling in chest, 1 of 8 with chest tightness, 7 of 11 with nasal symptoms, 6 of 11 with eye symptoms, and 3 of 4 with skin symptoms.

Eight (33%) participants noted that there was something at the facility that brought on chest symptoms. When asked what specifically brought on the chest symptoms, participants cited dust, compounds in the printweigh room, starch, flavorings, and soy flour. Seven (29%) participants noted that during the past 12 months, there was something at the facility that brought on nasal symptoms. When asked what specifically brought on the nasal symptoms, participants cited dust, starch, SAPP, sodium diacetate, and soy flour. Seven (29%) participants noted that during the past 12 months, there was something at the facility that brought on eye symptoms. When asked what specifically brought on the eye symptoms, participants cited dust, flavorings, SAPP, enrichment product, soy flour, and cleaning with compressed air. Four (17%) participants noted that there was something at the facility that brought on skin symptoms. When asked what specifically brought on the skin symptoms, participants cited enrichment product and compounds and chemicals in the printweigh room.

Four (17%) participants reported ever receiving a physician's diagnosis of asthma; one (4%) participant reported current physician-diagnosed asthma, which did not have a work-related pattern. Ten (42%) participants met the definition of asthma-like symptoms; 2 of these described work-related asthma-like symptoms. No participant reported a diagnosis of chronic bronchitis or emphysema.

Twenty-three (56%) employees underwent baseline spirometry testing, including 18 (67%) production workers. Twenty-two of the baseline spirometry tests were interpretable. Of these, 18 (82%) were interpreted as normal. Four (18%) were interpreted as having a restrictive pattern. None was interpreted as having an obstructive pattern. One (5%) of the post-bronchodilator tests showed a significant response to bronchodilator, in a worker with a restrictive pattern.

Of the four participants with restrictive pattern on spirometry, two had a mild restrictive pattern, one had a moderate restrictive pattern, and one had a moderately severe restrictive pattern. The participants with moderate and moderately severe restrictive patterns both reported respiratory symptoms.

Table 5 shows the PRs comparing General Mills participants with the U.S. adult population. The prevalences of shortness of breath when hurrying on level ground or walking up a slight hill, ever received a physician's diagnosis of asthma, and restrictive pattern on spirometry among General Mills participants were statistically significantly higher than the corresponding prevalences for the U.S. adult population.

We found no statistical association between shortness of breath when hurrying on level ground or walking up a slight hill, asthma-like symptoms, ever received a physician's diagnosis of asthma, a restrictive pattern on spirometry and participants' work experiences. Specifically, there was no association between these health outcomes and reported use of powdered flavorings, liquid flavorings, or flour; job title (mixer, packer, and printweigh vs. all other jobs); or length of tenure at General Mills.

Industrial Hygiene Survey

Real-Time VOC Air Concentrations

Airborne total VOC concentrations during real-time air sampling were variable by process. During the first industrial hygiene survey, for example, the average VOC concentration over a full shift (455 minutes) in the kitchen was 4.2 parts per billion (ppb); the peak measurement during the same time interval was 600 ppb. In contrast, the average concentration for a sample collected over a period of 454 minutes in Mixing (Line 2) during production of the re-formulated buttermilk cake doughnut mix was 26 ppb; the peak measurement was 2,000 ppb. Although the VOC concentration was 0 ppb in the QRO technician's breathing zone during preparation of the re-formulated buttermilk flavoring in the ingredients lab, concentrations ranged from 0 to 700 ppb during cleaning of equipment in a sink using warm water. The peak VOC concentration while the mixer operator poured re-formulated flavoring into the heated shortening tank was 19,703 ppb or 19.7 parts per million (ppm).

Ketones Identified in Bulk Samples

Table 6 provides semi-quantitative sampling data identifying ketone compounds in all bulk samples. Analysis of the re-formulated liquid buttermilk flavoring identified the following ketone compounds: diacetyl, acetoin, 2,3-pentanedione, 2,3-hexanedione, and 2-3, heptanedione; the predominant compound was 2,3-pentanedione. One or more of the same compounds were identified in all four powdered buttermilk flavorings, nutmeg oil, and the cake doughnut mix that contained the re-formulated liquid buttermilk flavoring.

Ketones Identified in Air

Table 7 provides semi-quantitative sampling data identifying ketone compounds detected in daily air samples collected from different areas of the facility using thermal desorption tubes. Diacetyl, acetoin, 2,3-pentanedione, 2,3-hexanedione, and 2,3-heptanedione were detected in air during batch preparation of the re-formulated buttermilk flavoring and during production of the cake doughnut mix. During these activities, 2,3-pentanedione was the predominant ketone compound.

Average Ketone Air Concentrations

During the first industrial hygiene survey, personal and area air concentrations of ketones (diacetyl and acetoin) were measured using Modified Occupational Safety and Health Administration (OSHA) Method PV2118 and are presented in Table 8. We collected personal air samples from nine workers, one during batch preparation of the re-formulated buttermilk flavoring and clean-up activities (duration < 90 min), and the remaining samples over an entire shift. Ten area air samples were collected, most concurrent with personal air samples. Results for all personal and area samples were less than the minimum detectable concentrations (MDCs) for diacetyl (47 ppb) and acetoin (93 ppb) in air.

During the second industrial hygiene survey, personal and area concentrations of ketones (diacetyl, acetoin, 2,3-pentanedione, 2,3-hexanedione, and 2,3-heptanedione) were measured using OSHA Method 1013 and are presented in Table 9. We collected personal air samples from 13 workers, one during batch preparation of the re-formulated buttermilk flavoring. Area air samples were collected in seven different work areas, many concurrent with the personal samples. Production of the cake doughnut mix began at approximately 10:00 AM (mid-shift) on May 27; therefore, all samples on that day were collected during the second half of the first shift (roughly 10:00 AM to 2:00 PM) and during the first half of the second shift (roughly 2:00 PM to 6:00 PM). All personal and area sampling results were less than the MDCs for diacetyl (24 ppb), acetoin (23 ppb), 2,3-hexanedione (14 ppb), and 2,3-heptanedione (6.4 ppb). One personal air sample collected from a first-shift packer resulted in 91 ppb for 2,3-pentanedione; the corresponding area air sample was 78 ppb for 2,3-pentanedione. Results of several other samples collected in the production room (mixing and packing) were between the MDC (20 ppb) and the minimum quantifiable concentration (MQC, 69 ppb) for 2,3-pentanedione.

Also during the second industrial hygiene survey, air concentrations of ketones (diacetyl, 2,3-pentanedione, 2,3-hexanedione, and 2,3-heptanedione) were measured using NIOSH Draft Procedure SMP2 and are presented in Table 10. Using this draft NIOSH procedure, only area air samples were collected and were concurrent with the area samples collected using OSHA Method 1013. Results of all samples analyzed using the procedure were less than the MDCs for diacetyl (2.4 ppb), 2,3-hexanedione (5.4 ppb), and 2,3-heptanedione (3.2 ppb); however, results of nearly all of the samples collected in the production room (mixing and packing) exceeded the MQC for 2,3-pentanedione (22 ppb); those that did exceed the MQC ranged from 48 to 95 ppb. The result of the sample collected on packing line during first shift was 95 ppb for 2,3-pentanedione (the corresponding sample collected using OSHA Method 1013 resulted in 78 ppb for pentanedione). Results were less than the MDC for 2,3-pentanedione (6.1 ppb) in the ingredients room, kitchen, and front offices.

Additionally, two air samples were collected during the second industrial hygiene survey using specially prepared, evacuated Silonite™ coated canisters (Entech Instruments, Inc., Simi Valley, CA). Both canister samples were collected alongside samples collected using the OSHA Method 1013 and the NIOSH Draft Procedure SMP2. Each was analyzed for diacetyl and 2,3-pentanedione. Resulting air concentrations collected during batch preparation of the re-formulated buttermilk flavoring were 25 ppb and 113 ppb for diacetyl and 2,3-pentanedione, respectively. Concentrations collected near the shortening tank during production of the cake doughnut mix were 23 ppb and 50 ppb for diacetyl and 2,3-pentanedione, respectively.

Average Aldehyde Air Concentrations

Personal and area air concentrations of aldehydes (acetaldehyde, benzaldehyde, and valeraldehyde) are presented in Table 8. Five personal air samples resulted in measurable concentrations of acetaldehyde (range = 9 to 18 ppb), benzaldehyde (range < MDC to 0.7 ppb), and valeraldehyde (range < MDC to 5.3 ppb). MDCs of acetaldehyde, benzaldehyde, and valeraldehyde were 0.46 ppb, 0.24 ppb, and 0.24 ppb, respectively. The sample resulting in the highest concentration of acetaldehyde (18 ppb), but non-detectable values of benzaldehyde and valeraldehyde, was from the QRO technician during short-duration batch preparation of the re-formulated liquid buttermilk flavoring. Ten area air samples also resulted in measurable concentrations of aldehydes: acetaldehyde (range = 7 to 15 ppb), benzaldehyde (range < MDC to 0.8 ppb), and valeraldehyde (range = 0.5 to 2.4 ppb). The highest concentration of acetaldehyde (15 ppb) was collected outside the ventilation hood in the ingredients lab during short-duration batch preparation of the re-formulated liquid buttermilk flavoring.

Respirable Particulate Air Concentrations

Personal and area time-weighted average (TWA) air concentrations of respirable dusts are presented in Table 8. Six personal and nine area air samples resulted in measurable respirable dust concentrations. The MDC was 0.037 mg/m³. Personal sample results ranged from 0.044 mg/m³ (Mixer, Line 2) to 0.292 mg/m³ (Printweigh worker). Area sample results ranged from < MDC (Palletizing) to 0.102 mg/m³ (Mixing, Line 2).

Of six real-time samples collected for airborne dust, the minimum average concentration was 0.004 mg/m³, collected in the palletizing work area. The maximum average concentration was 0.384 mg/m³ collected in Mixing (Line 2) during production of buttermilk cake doughnut mix. Peak concentrations were less than 5 mg/m³ in all production work areas, ranging from 0.195 mg/m³ in palletizing to 4.99 mg/m³ in the printweigh room.

Applicable OSHA PELs and NIOSH RELs

Respirable dust concentrations measured by NIOSH were well below the 5 mg/m³ TWA OSHA permissible exposure limit (PEL) for the respirable fraction of particulates not otherwise regulated (PNOR). Mineral, inorganic, or organic dusts not specifically listed by substance name, are covered by the PNOR limit; however, the absence of specific regulation does not imply safety. The OSHA PEL for PNOR applies to particulates with low toxicity and is not designed to protect workers from bronchiolitis obliterans or other chronic obstructive respiratory disorders.

Of the analytes measured by NIOSH, only acetaldehyde has an OSHA PEL and/or NIOSH recommended exposure limit (REL). All acetaldehyde exposures were below the OSHA PEL of 200 ppm TWA. NIOSH recommends the lowest exposure feasible for acetaldehyde because it is a potential carcinogen. Animal studies have shown nasal tumors in rats (Woutersen et al. 1986) and laryngeal tumors in hamsters (Feron et al. 1982) exposed to acetaldehyde.

Ventilation / Air Movement

In general, ventilation systems appeared to function adequately. We evaluated the ventilated hood in the ingredients lab where batch preparation of liquid flavorings took place. Smoke tubes indicated that the hood functioned appropriately by capturing all smoke released from just outside the hood opening.

We evaluated total VOC concentrations while batches of the re-formulated buttermilk flavoring were poured into the shortening tank in the production area. During the first industrial hygiene survey, the measured VOC concentration at the lid-tank interface was 22 ppm. Following the first survey, NIOSH recommended that a better seal between the shortening tank and lid would reduce volatile flavor chemical emissions into the general workplace air. Prior to the second industrial hygiene survey, General Mills added a rubber gasket at the interface, with metal clamps to ensure a better seal. During the second survey, total concentrations at the lid-tank interface were below detectable limits.

CONCLUSIONS

Our investigation found that in the past, some General Mills workers used a liquid buttermilk flavoring reported to contain 15-20% diacetyl under conditions that may have resulted in exposure. In addition, powered buttermilk flavorings containing a lower concentration (up to 1%) of diacetyl have been and continue to be used at the facility. In past investigations of workplaces that make or use flavorings containing diacetyl, some workers with the finding of fixed obstruction on spirometry had bronchiolitis obliterans, a rare, irreversible lung disease [CDC 2002; Akpinar-Elci et al. 2004; CDC 2007]. The lack of fixed obstruction on spirometry among the General Mills workers who participated in our medical survey indicates that they are very unlikely to have bronchiolitis obliterans. While many of the participants reported working with liquid or powered buttermilk flavorings, their generally infrequent use and existing exposure controls may have served to limit cumulative exposures.

A re-formulated liquid buttermilk flavoring was introduced at the facility in mid-2008. We found that the major substitute for diacetyl in this re-formulated flavoring is 2,3-pentanedione. The re-formulated flavoring also contains diacetyl; acetoin and acetoin derivatives; 2,3-hexanedione; and 2,3-heptanedione. The MSDS for this re-formulated flavoring listed only acetoin as a hazardous ingredient (percentage not shown), and did not list any other chemical constituents. All of these compounds are ketones, with the common characteristic among them being a carbon-oxygen double bond functional group. Diacetyl (or 2,3-butanedione) and acetoin are characterized by a four-carbon chain; 2,3-pentanedione, a five-carbon chain; 2,3-hexanedione, a six-carbon chain; and 2,3-heptanedione, a seven-carbon chain. We detected diacetyl, acetoin, 2,3-pentanedione, 2,3-hexanedione, and 2,3-heptanedione in the air in some areas during batch preparation of the re-formulated buttermilk flavoring and during production of the cake doughnut mix. The most commonly detected of these ketones was 2,3-pentanedione. While in most cases, the concentrations of these ketones were too low to be determined, we were able to determine concentrations of 2,3-pentanedione for a packer and the packing area.

The risks of exposure to diacetyl have been demonstrated through workplace investigations and laboratory-based studies [Kanwal et al. 2006; van Rooy et al. 2007; Hubbs et al. 2008]. A "safe" level of diacetyl has not been established, and even low levels of diacetyl are potentially hazardous. The toxicology of other flavoring ingredients, including diacetyl substitutes, is poorly described. Because 2,3-pentanedione, 2,3-hexanedione, and 2,3-heptanedione all share the same functional alpha-diketone group as diacetyl, these compounds may also share diacetyl's mechanism of toxicity. Indeed, the increasing carbon chain length would be predicted to reduce water solubility and result in deeper lung penetration and perhaps greater toxicity. Until more is known about 2,3-pentanedione and other alpha-diketone compounds, they should not be assumed to be safe.

The prevalence of a restrictive pattern on spirometry among General Mills participants was significantly higher than the prevalence for the U.S. adult population. While a restrictive pattern can be seen with a number of conditions, including obesity and respiratory muscle weakness, it may indicate the presence of lung disease, such as lung scarring or fibrosis. Further evaluation by a physician would be necessary to determine if participants with a restrictive pattern on spirometry have lung disease; recommendations for follow-up were provided to individual participants. We sought but were unable to obtain any results of recommended follow-up medical evaluations for those with restrictive patterns on spirometry and respiratory symptoms. While the significance of restrictive lung disease among flavorings-exposed workers is uncertain, NIOSH has received reports of restrictive lung disease in people who work with flavorings [Kreiss 2007], suggesting that the spectrum of health effects related to flavorings may be broader than fixed obstruction.

We are unable to make conclusions about the lung function of current General Mills employees who did not participate in spirometry testing, or about the lung function of former General Mills employees. Confirmation of an absence of lung disease among non-participants and former production employees would provide useful information about the risk of flavorings in food production.

Participants had higher than expected prevalence of shortness of breath hurrying on level ground or walking up a slight hill and of ever having received a physician's diagnosis of asthma compared to U.S. adults. While the prevalence of having a current asthma diagnosis was not elevated, 40% of the participants reported recent asthma-like symptoms. Our administration of bronchodilator did not document untreated asthma-like conditions, and interpretation of significant bronchodilator response in the context of a restrictive pattern is unclear. Elevated rates of respiratory problems among General Mills workers do not, by themselves, necessarily indicate a workplace cause, and we did not find statistical associations between health outcomes and work experiences (such as reported exposures, job title, or tenure). However, it is important to note that some participants had symptoms that improved away from work, indicating a work-related pattern. Such a pattern implicates the workplace as causing a work-related condition or exacerbating a non-work-related condition. Two of the 10 participants with asthma-like symptoms reported that those symptoms improved away from work. In addition, some participants reported cough or nose, eye, or skin symptoms with a work-related pattern. Work-related symptoms were most commonly attributed to dust, starch, and soy flour. Such symptoms may represent allergy to bakery antigens, such as flours and alpha-amylase. While average respirable dust levels were well below the OSHA PEL, peak levels in some areas, such as in the printweigh room, approached the OSHA PEL. In addition, we did not sample dust levels during some tasks, such as cleaning with compressed air, that may have resulted in higher dust concentrations. Thus, there was some evidence that adverse health outcomes among General Mills workers are related to workplace exposures; the small number of participants may have limited our ability to detect statistical associations between health outcomes and work experiences.

RECOMMENDATIONS

Based on our findings, we recommend the actions listed below to create a more healthful workplace. We encourage General Mills to use a labor-management health and safety committee or working group to discuss the recommendations in this report and develop an action plan. Those involved in the work can best set priorities and assess the feasibility of our recommendations for the specific situation at General Mills. Our recommendations are based on the hierarchy of controls approach. This approach groups actions by their likely effectiveness in reducing or removing hazards. In most cases, the preferred approach is to eliminate hazardous materials or processes and install engineering controls to reduce exposure or shield employees. Until such controls are in place, or if they are not effective or feasible, administrative measures and/or PPE may be needed.

Many of these recommendations were previously shared with General Mills in interim letters dated November 3, 2008 and March 31, 2009.

1. **Substitution:**

   General Mills took steps in 2008 to replace a flavoring reported to contain 15-20% diacetyl with a safer flavoring. Beyond acetoin, the re-formulated flavoring's principal flavoring ingredients were not identified on the MSDS or known to company safety representatives. The re-formulated flavoring has several alpha-diketones that may be as hazardous as diacetyl. Accordingly, substitution may not have its intended effect.

2. **Engineering controls:**

   Continue batch preparation of liquid flavoring chemicals inside the ventilated hood located in the ingredients room.

   Ensure that workers are trained on the operation and use of ventilation systems for reducing flavoring chemical exposures.

   Ensure that the seal at the shortening tank-lid interface is secured after pouring liquid flavorings into the tank.

3. **Respiratory protection:**

   Continue the required use of half-facepiece negative-pressure respirators with organic vapor cartridges during flavoring transfers in the ingredients room and during cleanup activities in the laboratory sink.

Instruct workers to use N-95 filtering-facepiece or half-face respirators with particulate filters when performing tasks that generate dust.

Continue to maintain a formal respiratory protection program that adheres to the requirements of the OSHA Respiratory Protection Standard (29 CFR 1910.134). The administrator for the program must have adequate training and experience to run it and regularly evaluate its effectiveness. The respiratory protection program must include a written policy, change-out schedule for canisters and cartridges, pre-use medical evaluation, pre-use and annual fit-testing and training, and the establishment and implementation of procedures for proper respirator use (such as prohibiting use with facial hair, ensuring a user seal check, inspection of respirators prior to each use, and ensuring proper storage of respirators to protect them from damage, contamination, dust, sunlight, and extreme temperatures). Details on the Respiratory Protection Standard and on how a company can set up a respiratory protection program are available on the OSHA website (http://www.osha.gov/SLTC/respiratoryprotection/index.html).

4. **Medical surveillance:**

   With input from the IBT union representative, establish procedures for workers to report symptoms to management. The establishment of these procedures should include designating an individual at the workplace to whom workers should report symptoms. Encourage workers to report new, persistent, or worsening symptoms to their personal physician and to this designated individual at the workplace. Reports of such symptoms should prompt investigation, which could include using employee health questionnaires to collect information on symptoms and reconsideration of measures to limit exposures. Workers with work-related upper airway or asthma symptoms may benefit from evaluation for allergy to bakery antigens, e.g., soy, wheat, and alpha-amylase.

   It is important to note that workers with flavoring-related lung disease may not have symptoms early in the course of their illness, and symptoms that are due to flavoring-related lung disease may not have a work-related pattern [NIOSH 2004]. Thus we recommend that in addition to a system for symptom reporting, General Mills consider the use of serial spirometry to detect declines in lung function that may be due to flavorings. While none of the participants tested in the NIOSH medical survey had obstruction on spirometry, and the recent introduction of ingredient substitution, engineering controls, and respiratory protection at the plant has likely reduced exposures to diacetyl, the toxicology of diacetyl substitutes, most notably 2,3-pentanedione, is unknown. Preliminary impressions presented by Daniel Morgan of the National Institute of Environmental Health Sciences at the 2009 Professional Conference on Industrial Hygienist were that 2,3-pentanedione has toxicity similar to diacetyl's toxicity in rodents. Serial spirometry, performed at baseline and at least annually [NIOSH 2004], could be used to confirm that interventions intended to limit exposures to flavoring chemicals have been successful in preventing declines in lung function. If over time, serial spirometry does not detect abnormal declines in lung function among exposed workers and exposure conditions do not change, it would then be reasonable to forego further serial spirometry. If symptomatic restriction is documented, it would be prudent to ensure that affected workers receive pulmonary consultation for evaluation of possible work-related lung disease, particularly for diagnoses associated with bioaerosol exposures in this industry.

5. **Work practices:**

   Liquid flavoring chemical containers handled outside the ventilation hood in the ingredients room should be closed to prevent the release of volatile chemicals into room air.

   Keep all tanks and containers of flavoring chemicals / ingredients sealed at all possible times.

   Maintain and use volatile flavoring chemicals at the lowest temperature possible according to the manufacturers' recommendations.

   Continue the use of cold water (versus hot), when feasible, during cleanup activities to minimize the volatization of flavoring chemicals.

Add flavoring ingredients into a tank last, when possible, to minimize the time during which vapors can enter the room air when the tank is open.

Clean spills promptly to minimize emissions of chemical vapors. Wear PPE, including respirators (with organic vapor cartridges and particulate filters) and eye and skin protection, when cleaning up spills or when washing empty containers or plant equipment that has been in contact with flavoring chemicals or ingredients. If any flavoring chemicals are disposed of via floor or sink drains, flush the drains immediately with water to minimize the potential for any chemical vapors to be released back into production rooms. Clean powder spills using vacuum cleaners equipped with HEPA filters.

Instead of using compressed air in blowdowns or dry-brushing or dry-sweeping, use vacuum cleaners equipped with HEPA filters as much as possible to clean residual powders from equipment.

6. **Skin protection:**

   Provide workers with appropriate protective clothing, gloves, and eye protection to prevent skin or eye contact with flavoring chemicals.

   If hands or other areas of the body with exposed skin contact flavoring chemicals, promptly wash with soap and water.

7. **Administrative controls:**

   Limit entry into production rooms and laboratories to production or laboratory workers and supervisory staff only.

   Structure work tasks to minimize time spent in proximity to flavoring chemicals and production processes with these chemicals.

   When flavoring chemical use is not enclosed or contained, workers in the vicinity of others handling flavoring chemicals must be informed and required to use appropriate PPE to prevent standby exposures.

8. Labeling containers and posting of work areas

Clearly label containers with flavoring chemicals and post signs in areas where these chemicals will be used or stored.

Post warning labels and signs describing the health risks associated with flavoring chemical exposures at entrances to work areas and inside work areas where airborne concentration of diacetyl, or other flavoring chemicals, may be present.

Depending on work practices and the airborne concentrations of diacetyl or other flavoring chemicals, post warning labels and signs describing the need for PPE in the work area. If respiratory protection is required, post the statement: "Respiratory Protection Required in this Area."

References

Akpinar-Elci M, Travis WD, Lynch DA, Kreiss K. [2004]. Bronchiolitis obliterans syndrome in popcorn production plant workers. Eur Respir J. 24(2):298-302.

Brant A [2007]. Baker's asthma. Curr Opin Allergy Clin Immunol. 7(2):152-155.

Centers for Disease Control and Prevention (CDC) [1996]. Third National Health and Nutrition Examination Survey, 1988–1994, NHANES III Laboratory Data File. Hyattsville, MD: National Center for Health Statistics (NCHS) Public use data file documentation no. 76200 (CD ROM).

Centers for Disease Control and Prevention (CDC) [2002]. Fixed obstructive lung disease in workers at a microwave popcorn factory–Missouri, 2000-2002. MMWR Morb Mortal Wkly Rep. 51(16):345-347.

Centers for Disease Control and Prevention (CDC) [2007]. Fixed obstructive lung disease among workers in the flavor-manufacturing industry–California, 2004-2007. MMWR Morb Mortal Wkly Rep. 56(16):389-393.

Ferris BG [1978]. Epidemiology standardization project. Am Rev Respir Dis. 108:1-113.

Feron VJ, Kruysse A, Woutersen RA [1982]. Respiratory tract tumours in hamsters exposed to acetaldehyde vapour alone or simultaneously to benzo(a)pyrene or diethylnitrosamine. Eur J Cancer Clin Oncol. 18(l):13-31.

Grassi M, Rezzani C, Biino G, Marinoni A [2003]. Asthma-like symptoms assessment through ECRHS screening questionnaire scoring. J Clin Epidemiol. 56(3):238-247.

Hankinson JL, Odencrantz JR, Fedan KB [1999]. Spirometric reference values from a sample of the general U.S. population. Am J Respir Crit Care Med. 159:179-187.

Hubbs AF. Goldsmith WT, Kashon ML, Frazer D, Mercer RR, Battelli LA, Kullman GJ, Schwegler-Berry D, Friend S, Castranova V. [2008]. Respiratory toxicologic pathology of inhaled diacetyl in Sprague-Dawley rats. Toxicol Pathol. 36(2):330-344.

Kanwal R, Kullman G, Piacitelli C, Boylstein R, Sahakian N, Martin S, Fedan K, Kreiss K [2006]. Evaluation of flavorings-related lung disease risk at six microwave popcorn plants. J Occup Environ Med. 48(2):149-157.

Kreiss K, Gomaa A, Kullman G, Fedan K, Simoes EJ, Enright PL [2002]. Clinical bronchiolitis obliterans in workers at a microwave-popcorn plant. N Engl J Med. 347(5):330-338.

Kreiss K [2007]. Flavoring-related bronchiolitis obliterans. Curr Opin Allergy Clin Immunol. 7(2):162-167.

Miller MR, Hankinson J, Brusasco V, Burgos F, Casaburi R, Coates A, Crapo R, Enright P, van der Grinten CP, Gustafsson P, Jensen R, Johnson DC, MacIntyre N, McKay R, Navajas D, Pedersen OF, Pellegrino R, Viegi G, Wanger J [2005]. ATS/ERS Task Force. Standardisation of spirometry. Eur Respir J. 26(2):319-338.

National Institute for Occupational Safety and Health (NIOSH) [2003]. In: Schlecht P, O'Connor P, eds. Manual of Analytical Methods (NMAM), 4th ed., Third Supplement. Cincinnati, OH: U.S. Department of Health and Human Services, DHHS (NIOSH) Publication No. 2003-154.

National Institute for Occupational Safety and Health (NIOSH) [2004]. NIOSH Alert: Preventing lung disease in workers that use or make flavorings. Division of Respiratory Disease Studies, National Institute for Occupational Safety and Health, Department of Health and Human Services, DHHS (NIOSH) Publication Number 2004-110.

National Institute for Occupational Safety and Health (NIOSH) [2008]. Health Hazard Evaluation and Technical Assistance Report: Gold Coast Ingredients, Inc., Commerce, California. Morgantown, WV: U.S. Department of Health and Human Services, Public Health Service, Centers for Disease Control, National Institute for Occupational Safety and Health, DHHS (NIOSH) Publication No. 2007-0033-3074.

Occupational Safety and Health Administration (OSHA). [September 2008]. Method 1013, Acetoin and Diacetyl. Accessible from: http://www.osha.gov/dts/sltc/methods/validated/1013/1013.html.

Parmet AJ, Von Essen S [2002]. Rapidly progressive, fixed airway obstructive disease in popcorn workers: a new occupational pulmonary illness? J Occup Environ Med. 44(3):216-218.

Pellegrino R, Viegi G, Brusasco V, Crapo RO, Burgos F, Casaburi R, Coates A, van der Grinten CP, Gustafsson P, Hankinson J, Jensen R, Johnson DC, MacIntyre N, McKay R, Miller MR, Navajas D, Pedersen OF, Wanger JJ[2005]. Interpretative strategies for lung function tests. Eur Respir J. 26(5):948-968.

van Rooy FG, Rooyackers JM, Prokop M, Houba R, Smit LA, Heederik DJ [2007]. Bronchiolitis obliterans syndrome in chemical workers producing diacetyl for food flavorings. Am J Respir Crit Care Med. 176(5):498-504.

Woutersen RA, Appelman LM, Van Garderen-Hoetmer A, Feron VJ [1986]. Inhalation toxicity of acetaldehyde in rats. III. Carcinogenicity study. Toxicology 41:213-231.

TABLES

Table 1. Sampling and analytical methods used during the September-October 2008 survey at General Mills.

Analytes	Media/sampler	Flow Rate (L/min)	Sample Duration (min)	Analytical Method	Objective
Volatile organic chemicals (VOCs) in bulks	Thermal desorption tube	0.1	1 (liquid) 30 (powder)	Gas chromatography / mass spectrometry by NIOSH headspace analysis	Screening for identification
Ketones in air (diacetyl, acetoin)	Sorbent tubes (silica gel 200mg/400mg)	0.05	240 x 2	Gas chromatography by Modified OSHA PV2118	Time-weighted average (TWA) concentrations
Aldehydes in air (acetaldehyde, benzaldehyde, valeraldehyde)	Sorbent tube (silica gel treated with 2,4 dinitrophenyl-hydrazine)	0.1	480	High performance liquid chromatography by NOISH 2016	TWA concentrations
Respirable dust in air	37-mm PVC filter with cyclone	1.7	480	Gravimetric analysis by NIOSH 0600	TWA concentrations
Volatile organic chemicals (VOCs) in air	Thermal desorption tube	0.02	480	Gas chromatography / mass spectrometry by NIOSH 2549	Screening for identification
Real-time VOCs in air	Photo-ionization detector (PID) ppbRAE Plus®	0.4	Variable	Direct-reading instruments (Rae Systems, Inc., Sunnyvale, CA)	TWA, continuous, and spot measurements
Real-time VOCs in air	PID ToxiRAE Plus®	0 (Passive)	Variable	Direct-reading instruments (Rae Systems, Inc., Sunnyvale, CA)	TWA, continuous, and spot measurements
Real-time respirable dust in air	Photometric meter, PersonalData RAM® pDR-1000AN	0 (Passive)	Variable	Direct-reading instrument (Thermo Electron Corporation, Franklin, MA)	TWA, continuous, and spot measurements

Table 2. Sampling and analytical methods used during the May 2009 survey at General Mills.

Analytes	Media/sampler	Flow Rate (L/min)	Sample Duration (min)	Analytical Method	Objective
Ketones in air (diacetyl, acetoin, 2,3-pentanedione, 2,3-hexane-dione, 2,3-heptanedione)	Sorbent tubes (silica gel 200mg/400mg)	0.05	240 x 2	Gas chromatography by OSHA Method 1013*	Time-weighted average (TWA) concentrations
Ketones in air (diacetyl, 2,3-pentanedione, 2,3-hexane-dione, 2,3-heptanedione)	Sorbent tubes (silica gel treated with o-phenylene-diamine)	0.05	240 x 2	Gas chromatography by NIOSH Draft Procedure SMP2	Time-weighted average (TWA) concentrations
Ketones in air (diacetyl, 2,3-pentanedione)	Silonite™ coated canisters (6L)	0.08 and 0.02	51 and 410	Gas chromatography- Mass spectrometry	Time-weighted average (TWA) concentrations
Volatile organic chemicals (VOCs) in air	Thermal desorption tube	0.02	480	Gas chromatography / mass spectrometry by NIOSH 2549	Screening for identification
Real-time VOCs in air	Photo-ionization detector (PID) ppbRAE Plus®	0.4	Variable	Direct-reading instruments (Rae Systems, Inc., Sunnyvale, CA)	TWA, continuous, and spot measurements
Real-time VOCs in air	PID ToxiRAE Plus®	0 (Passive)	Variable	Direct-reading instruments (Rae Systems, Inc., Sunnyvale, CA)	TWA, continuous, and spot measurements

*OSHA Method 1013 is fully validated for diacetyl and acetoin, but not for 2,3-pentanedione, 2,3-hexanedione, or 2,3-heptanedione.

Table 3. Frequency of working with flour and buttermilk flavorings among 24 participants.

	Flour	Buttermilk Flavorings	
		Powdered	Liquid
	No. (%)	No. (%)	No. (%)
General Mills facility			
Ever	23 (96)	18 (75)	12 (50)
Never	1 (4)	6 (25)	12 (50)
Current job			
Daily	14 (58)	2 (8)	0
Weekly	1 (4)	2 (8)	4 (17)
Monthly	0	6 (25)	3 (13)
Less than monthly	1 (4)	2 (8)	1 (4)
Never	8 (33)	12 (50)	16 (67)

Table 4. Chest, nasal, eye, and skin symptoms among 24 General Mills participants.

Symptom	No. (%)
Usual cough	4 (17)
Shortness of breath	
Hurrying on level ground or walking up a slight hill	10 (42)
Walking with people of own age on level ground	4 (17)
Wheezing or whistling in chest*	5 (21)
Woken up with feeling of tightness in chest*	8 (33)
Stuffy, itchy, runny nose*	11 (46)
Watery, itchy eyes*	11 (46)
New skin rash or skin problems[†]	4 (17)

* During the past 12 months
[†] Since began working at the General Mills facility

Table 5. Comparison of respiratory symptoms, diagnoses, and spirometry findings among General Mills participants with US adults (NHANES III).

Symptom, diagnosis, or spirometry finding	PR	95% CI
Usual cough on most days for 3 consecutive months or more	1.7	0.5-6.1
Shortness of breath hurrying on level ground/walking up slight hill	2.1	1.1-4.1
Wheezing or whistling in chest*	1.9	0.8-4.5
Stuffy, itchy, runny nose*	1.1	0.6-2.1
Watery, itchy eyes*	1.3	0.7-2.4
Ever asthma[†]	3.6	1.4-9.3
Current asthma[†]	1.4	0.2-7.9
Restrictive pattern on spirometry	2.9	1.1-7.5

NHANES III, Third National Health and Nutrition Examination Survey; PR, Prevalence ratio; CI, Confidence interval
* During the past 12 months
[†] Physician-diagnosed

Table 6. Ketone compounds in bulk samples (measured with thermal desorption tubes).

Bulk Samples	Manufacturer	Diacetyl	Acetoin	2,3-Pentanedione	2,3-Hexanedione	2,3-Heptanedione
Re-formulated liquid buttermilk flavoring	A	X	X[1]	X	X	X
Powdered buttermilk flavoring #1	B			X		X
Powdered buttermilk flavoring #2	C	X		X		
Powdered buttermilk flavoring #3	D	X	X	X		X
Powdered buttermilk flavoring #4	---[2]	X				
Nutmeg oil[3]	E[4]		X	X		

[1]Listed as a hazardous ingredient on the Material Safety Data Sheet (MSDS);
[2]Manufacturer unknown (no MSDS provided);
[3]Predominant chemicals included furfural, terpenes, and terpene derivatives;
[4]No MSDS provided.

Table 7. Ketone compounds in air (measured with thermal desorption tubes).
We collected a sample in the printweigh room on 9/30/08, but do not report results because the sample was likely contaminated prior to analysis.

Work Area/Process Description	Date Sampled	Diacetyl	Acetoin	2,3-Pentanedione	2,3-Hexanedione	2,3-Heptanedione
Ingredients lab (outside hood)[1]	9/30/08			X		
Ingredients lab (inside hood)[1]	9/30/08	X	X	X		X
Packing (Line 1)[2]	9/30/08			X		
Packing (Line 2)[3]	10/1/08	X		X	X	X
Mixing (near shortening tank)[3]	10/1/08	X		X	X	X
Palletizing[3]	10/1/08					
Ingredients lab (outside hood)[2]	10/2/08					
Mixing (between dump stations)[2]	10/2/08			X		
Printweigh room[4]	10/2/08					
Ingredients lab (outside hood)[1]	5/26/09			X		
Ingredients lab (inside hood)[1]	5/26/09	X		X	X	X
Mixing (between dump stations)[2,4]	5/27/09	X	X	X	X	X
Packing (Line 1)[2]	5/27/09			X		
Packing (Line 2)[3]	5/27/09	X	X	X	X	X
Mixing (near shortening tank)[3]	5/27/09	X	X	X	X	X
Kitchen[3]	5/27/09					
Front offices[2]	5/27/09					

[1]Batch preparation of re-formulated liquid buttermilk flavoring (task samples);
[2]Re-formulated liquid buttermilk flavoring not used in these areas/processes [a powdered buttermilk flavoring used on Packing (Line 1) on 9/30/08];
[3]Re-formulated liquid buttermilk flavoring used in these areas/processes;
[4]Upon analysis, flour and possibly other dry powdered ingredients observed inside sample tube.

Table 8. Air concentrations of ketones, aldehydes, and respirable dust by sample type and job or work area in the first industrial hygiene survey.

Sample Type	Job or Work Area	Date Sampled	Diacetyl (ppb)	Acetoin (ppb)	Acetaldehyde (ppb)	Benzaldehyde (ppb)	Valeraldehyde (ppb)	Respirable Dust (mg/m³)
Personal	QRO technician	9/30/08	<MDC[1]	<MDC	18	<MDC	<MDC	---
Area	Ingredients lab (inside hood)	9/30/08	<MDC	<MDC	---	---	---	---
Area	Ingredients lab (outside hood)	9/30/08	---[2]	---	15	<MDC	<MQC (2.0)	<MDC
Personal	Printweigh worker	9/30/08	<MDC	<MDC	---	---	---	---
Area	Printweigh room	9/30/08	<MDC	<MDC	9	<MQC[3] (0.4)	1.0	0.081
Personal	Mixer (Line 1)	9/30/08	<MDC	<MDC	---	---	---	---
Personal	Mixer (Line 2)	9/30/08	---	---	---	---	---	0.081
Personal	Packer (Line 1)	9/30/08	<MDC	<MDC	---	---	---	---
Area	Packing (Line 1)	9/30/08	<MDC	<MDC	10	<MQC (0.4)	0.9	0.068
Personal	Packer (Line 2)	9/30/08	---	---	---	---	---	0.047
Personal	Team leader	10/1/08	<MDC	<MDC	---	---	---	---
Personal	Mixer (Line 2)	10/1/08	<MDC	<MDC	9	<MQC (0.3)	<MQC (0.7)	0.102
Area	Mixing (near shortening tank)	10/1/08	<MDC	<MDC	11	<MQC (0.4)	1.0	0.010
Personal	Packer (Line 2)	10/1/08	<MDC	<MDC	---	---	---	---
Area	Packing (Line 2)	10/1/08	<MDC	---	9	<MQC (0.5)	0.9	0.125
Personal	Mixer (Line 1)	10/1/08	---	---	---	<MQC (0.4)	<MQC (0.8)	0.292
Personal	Packer (Line 1)	10/1/08	---	<MDC	---	---	---	---
Personal	Printweigh worker	10/1/08	<MDC	<MDC	---	---	---	<MDC
Personal	Palletizer operator	10/1/08	<MDC	<MDC	---	---	---	---
Area	Palletizing	10/1/08	<MDC	<MDC	7	<MQC (0.4)	<MQC (0.5)	---
Personal	QRO technician	10/1/08	---	---	14	<MQC (0.7)	5.3	0.056
Personal	QRO technician	10/2/08	<MDC	<MDC	---	---	---	0.044
Area	Kitchen	10/2/08	<MDC	<MDC	10	<MQC (0.8)	2.4	0.081
Personal	Mixer (Line 2)	10/2/08	---	---	---	---	---	---
Area	Mixing (between dump stations)	10/2/08	<MDC	<MDC	9	<MQC (0.6)	1.2	---
Personal	Packer (Line 1)	10/2/08	---	---	10	<MQC (0.3)	1.0	---
Personal	Printweigh worker	10/2/08	---	---	---	---	---	0.141
Area	Printweigh room	10/2/08	<MDC	<MDC	8	<MQC (0.5)	<MQC (0.6)	0.093
Area	Front offices	10/2/08	<MDC	<MDC	8	<MQC (0.4)	<MQC (0.6)	---

[1] MDC = Minimum detectable concentration in air; [2] ~ sample not collected;
[3] MQC = Minimum quantifiable concentration in air

Table 9. Air concentrations of ketones by sample type and job or work area in the second industrial hygiene survey (measured by OSHA Method 1013).

Sample Type	Job or Work Area	Date Sampled	Shift	Duration (min)	Diacetyl (ppb)	Acetoin (ppb)	2,3-Pentane-dione (ppb)	2,3-Hexane-dione (ppb)	2,3-Heptane-dione (ppb)
Area	Ingredients lab (outside hood)	5/26/09	1	53	< MDC[1]	<MDC	<MDC	<MDC	<MDC
Personal	QRO technician	5/26/09	1	58	<MDC	<MDC	<MDC	<MDC	<MDC
Area	Kitchen	5/27/09	1 & 2	448	<MDC	<MDC	<MDC	<MDC	<MDC
Area	Front offices	5/27/09	1 & 2	451	<MDC	<MDC	<MDC	<MDC	<MDC
Personal	Team leader	5/27/09	1	254	<MDC	<MDC	<MDC	<MDC	<MDC
Personal	Team leader	5/27/09	2	227	<MDC	<MDC	<MDC	<MDC	<MDC
Area	Packing (Line 1)	5/27/09	1	250	<MDC	<MDC	<MQC[2] (59)	<MDC	<MDC
Personal	Packer (Line 1)	5/27/09	1	245	<MDC	<MDC	<MQC (42)	<MDC	<MDC
Area	Packing (Line 1)	5/27/09	2	190	<MDC	<MDC	<MQC (51)	<MDC	<MDC
Personal	Packer (Line 1)	5/27/09	2	214	<MDC	<MDC	<MDC	<MDC	<MDC
Area	Packing (Line 2)	5/27/09	1	257	<MDC	<MDC	78	<MDC	<MDC
Personal	Packer (Line 2)	5/27/09	1	219	<MDC	<MDC	91	<MDC	<MDC
Area	Packing (Line 2)	5/27/09	2	192	<MDC	<MDC	<MQC (51)	<MDC	<MDC
Personal	Packer (Line 2)	5/27/09	2	206	<MDC	<MDC	<MQC (40)	<MDC	<MDC
Area	Mixing (between dump stations)	5/27/09	1	264	<MDC	<MDC	<MQC (56)	<MDC	<MDC
Personal	Mixer (Line 1)	5/27/09	1	128[3]	<MDC	<MDC	<MDC	<MDC	<MDC
Area	Mixing (between dump stations)	5/27/09	2	192	<MDC	<MDC	<MQC (56)	<MDC	<MDC
Personal	Mixer (Line 1)	5/27/09	2	210	<MDC	<MDC	<MDC	<MDC	<MDC
Area	Mixing (near shortening tank)	5/27/09	1	252	<MDC	<MDC	<MQC (48)	<MDC	<MDC
Personal	Mixer (Line 2)	5/27/09	1	248	<MDC	<MDC	<MQC (53)	<MDC	<MDC
Area	Mixing (near shortening tank)	5/27/09	2	188	<MDC	<MDC	<MDC	<MDC	<MDC
Personal	Mixer (Line 2)	5/27/09	2	179[3]	<MDC	<MDC	<MDC	<MDC	<MDC
Personal	Palletizer operator	5/27/09	1	121[3]	<MDC	<MDC	<MDC	<MDC	<MDC
Personal	Palletizer operator	5/27/09	2	207	<MDC	<MDC	<MDC	<MDC	<MDC

[1] MDC = Minimum detectable concentration in air
[2] MQC = Minimum quantifiable concentration in air
[3] faulty pump

Table 10. Air concentrations of ketones by work area in the second industrial hygiene survey (measured by Draft NIOSH Procedure SMP2).

Job or Work Area	Date Sampled	Shift	Duration (min)	Diacetyl (ppb)	2,3-Pentane-dione (ppb)	2,3-Hexane-dione (ppb)	2,3-Heptane-dione (ppb)
Ingredients lab (outside hood)	5/26/09	1	53	< MDC[1]	<MDC	<MDC	<MDC
Kitchen	5/27/09	1 & 2	447	<MDC	<MDC	<MDC	<MDC
Front offices	5/27/09	1 & 2	451	<MDC	<MDC	<MDC	<MDC
Packing (Line 1)	5/27/09	1	251	<MDC	62	<MDC	<MDC
Packing (Line 1)	5/27/09	2	190	<MDC	49	<MDC	<MDC
Packing (Line 2)	5/27/09	1	257	<MDC	95	<MDC	<MDC
Packing (Line 2)	5/27/09	2	193	<MDC	53	<MDC	<MDC
Mixing (between dump stations)	5/27/09	1	263	<MDC	56	<MDC	<MDC
Mixing (between dump stations)	5/27/09	2	193	<MDC	53	<MDC	<MDC
Mixing (near shortening tank)	5/27/09	1	253	<MDC	48	<MDC	<MDC
Mixing (near shortening tank)	5/27/09	2	189	<MDC	<MQC[2] (23)	<MDC	<MDC

[1] MDC = Minimum detectable concentration in air
[2] MQC = Minimum quantifiable concentration in air (based on the sampling duration, the MQC for 2,3-pentanedione in this sample was 28 ppb)

ID _____

HETA 2008 – 0230
General Mills
5469 Ferguson Drive
Los Angeles, CA

Interviewer: _____   Interview Date: __ __ / __ __ / __ __ __ __
                                                    (Month) (Day)   (Year)

Section I: Identification and Demographic Information

Name: _____ _____ ____
          (Last name)   (First name)   (MI)

Address: _____
              (Number, Street, and/or Rural Route)

_____ _____ _____
(City)   (State)   (Zip Code)

Home Telephone Number: (   ) _____ - _____

If you were to move, is there someone who would know how to contact you?

Name: _____ _____ ____
          (Last name)   (First name)   (MI)

Relationship to you: _____

Address: _____
              (Number, Street, and/or Rural Route)

_____ _____ _____
(City)   (State)   (Zip Code)

Home Telephone Number: (   ) _____ - _____

1. Date of Birth: __ __ / __ __ / __ __ __ __
                                            (Month) (Day)   (Year)

2. Sex: 1. ____ Male 2. ____ Female

3. Are you Spanish, Hispanic, or Latino?   1. ____ Yes 2. ____ No.

4. Select <u>one or more</u> of the following categories to describe your race:
                                            1. ___ American Indian or Alaska Native
                                            2. ___ Asian
                                            3. ___ African-American or Black
                                            4. ___ Native Hawaiian or Other Pacific Islander
                                            5. ___ White

ID _____

Section II: Health Information

I'm going to ask you some questions about your health. The answer to many of these questions will be "Yes" or "No." If you are in doubt about whether to answer "Yes" or "No," then please answer "No."

5.   During the last 12 months, have you had any trouble with your breathing?

                                                        1. ___ Yes   0. ___ No

IF YES:

> a) Which of the following statements best describes your breathing?
> 1._____I only rarely have trouble with my breathing.
> 2._____I have regular trouble with my breathing, but it always gets completely better.
> 3._____My breathing is never quite right.

6.   Do you usually have a cough?   1. ___ Yes   0. ___ No
     (Count cough with first smoke or on first going
     out-of-doors. Exclude clearing of throat.)

IF YES:

> a)   Do you usually cough on most days for 3
>   consecutive months or more during the year?   1. ___ Yes   0. ___ No
>
> b)   In what month and year did the cough begin?   __ __ / __ __ __ __
>   (Month)   (Year)
>
> c)   When you are away from this facility on days off or on vacation, is this cough:
>   1. ___ The same   2. ___ Better   3. ___ Worse

7.   Are you troubled by shortness of breath when hurrying
     on level ground or walking up a slight hill?   1. ___ Yes   0. ___ No

IF YES:

> a)   Do you get short of breath walking with people
>   of your own age on level ground?   1. ___ Yes   0. ___ No
>
> b)   Do you ever have to stop for breath when
>   walking at your own pace on level ground?   1. ___ Yes   0. ___ No
>
> c)   In what month and year did this breathlessness start?   __ __ / __ __ __ __
>   (Month)   (Year)

8. Have you had wheezing or whistling in your chest at any time in the last 12 months?

                                                         1. ___ Yes   0. ___ No

IF YES:

> a)   Have you been at all breathless when the wheezing noise was present?
>   1. ___ Yes   0. ___ No

ID _____

---

b) Have you had this wheezing or whistling when you did not have a cold?

1. ___ Yes   0. ___ No

c) In what month and year did this wheezing or whistling start?   __ __ / __ __ __ __
(Month)   (Year)

d) When you are away from this facility on days off or on vacation, is this wheezing or whistling
1. ____ The same   2. ____ Better   3. ____ Worse

---

9. Have you woken up with a feeling of tightness in your chest at any time in the last 12 months?

1. ___ Yes   0. ___ No

IF YES:

---

a) In what month and year did this chest tightness start?   __ __ / __ __ __ __
(Month)   (Year)

b) When you are away from this facility, on days off or on vacation, is this problem
1. ____ The same   2. ____ Better   3. ____ Worse

---

10. Have you had an attack of asthma in the last 12 months?

1. ___ Yes   0. ___ No

IF YES:

---

a) When you are away from this facility on days off or on vacation, is this problem
1. ____ The same   2. ____ Better   3. ____ Worse

---

11. Are you currently taking any medicine (including inhalers, aerosols, or tablets) for asthma?

1. ___ Yes   0. ___ No

IF YES:

---

a) When you are away from this facility on days off or on vacation, do you take the medicine for asthma:
1. ____ The same   2. ____ More often   3. ____ Less often

---

12. Is there anything at this facility that brings on chest symptoms, such as cough, shortness of breath, wheezing, or chest tightness?   1. ___ Yes   0. ___ No
IF YES:

---

a) What brings on these chest symptoms?

_____

_____

---

13. Have you ever had to change your job, job duties, or work area at this facility because of breathing difficulties?   1. ___ Yes   0. ___ No
IF YES:

---

a) What month and year did you change your job, job duties, or work area?   __ __ / __ __ __ __
(Month)   (Year)

ID _____

> b) What was your job, job duties, and/or work area before the change?
> Describe: _____
> _____
>
> c) How did your job, job duties, and/or work area differ after the change?
> Describe: _____
>
> d) Were your breathing problems after the change:
> 1. ____ The same   2. ____ Better   3. ____ Worse

14. Has a doctor <u>ever</u> told you that you had asthma?   1. ___ Yes   0. ___ No
IF YES:

> a) In what month and year were you first told that you had asthma?
> ___ ___ / ___ ___ ___ ___
> (Month)   (Year)
>
> b) Do you still have asthma?   1. ___ Yes   0. ___ No
>
> c) Did your asthma ever go away for at least a year, only to come back again?
> 1. ___ Yes   0. ___ No
>
> IF YES:
> d) In what month and year did your asthma come back?   ___ ___ / ___ ___ ___ ___
> (Month)   (Year)

15. Has a doctor <u>ever</u> told you that you had chronic bronchitis?   1. ___ Yes   0. ___ No
IF YES:

> a) Do you still have chronic bronchitis?   1. ___ Yes   0. ___ No
>
> b) In what month and year were you first told that you had chronic bronchitis ___ ___ / ___ ___ ___ ___
> (Month)   (Year)

16. Has a doctor <u>ever</u> told you that you had emphysema?   1. ___ Yes   0. ___ No
IF YES:

> a) Do you still have emphysema?   1. ___ Yes   0. ___ No
>
> b) In what month and year were you first told that you had emphysema ___ ___ / ___ ___ ___ ___
> (Month)   (Year)

17. Has a doctor <u>ever</u> told you that you had eczema?   1. ___ Yes   0. ___ No

18. Do you have any nasal allergies including hay fever?   1. ___ Yes   0. ___ No

19. During the past 12 months, have you had any episodes of stuffy, itchy, runny nose?
1. ___ Yes   0. ___ No

ID _____

IF YES:

a)   Is there anything at this facility that brings on these nasal symptoms?

1. ___ Yes   0. ___ No

IF YES:

b) What brings on these nasal symptoms?

_____

_____

c) In what month and year did these nasal symptoms start? __ __ / __ __ __ __

(Month)   (Year)

d) When you are away from work on days off or on vacation, are your nasal symptoms?

1. ___ The same   2. ___ Better   3. ___ Worse

20. During the past 12 months, have you had any episodes of watery, itchy eyes?

1. ___ Yes 0. ___ No

IF YES:

a)   Is there anything at this facility that brings on these eye symptoms?

1. ___ Yes   0. ___ No

IF YES:

b)   What brings on these eye symptoms?

_____

c) In what month and year did these eye symptoms start?   __ __ / __ __ __ __

(Month)   (Year)

d) When you are away from work on days off or on vacation, are your eye symptoms:

1. ___ The same   2. ___ Better   3. ___ Worse

21.   Since you began working at this facility, have you had any new skin rash or skin problems?

1. ___ Yes   0. ___ No

IF YES:

a)   Is there anything at this facility that brings on this skin rash or skin problem?

1. ___ Yes   0. ___ No

IF YES:

b) What brings on this skin rash or skin problem?

_____

_____

c) In what month and year did this skin rash or skin problem start? __ __ / __ __ __ __

(Month)   (Year)

d) When you are away from work on days off or on vacation, are these skin problems:

1. ___ The same   2. ___ Better   3. ___ Worse

22.   Is there anything else about your health, related to work, that concerns you?

ID _____

1. ___ Yes   0. ___ No

IF YES:
a) Describe your concerns:

_____

Section III. Work Information

I'm now going to ask you questions about your work history at this facility.

23.   During an average work week, how many hours do you work at this facility?

_____ Hours per week

I have some questions about all the jobs that you have had while at this facility. We will start with your current job and work back through time.

24.

Main Work Area (Production room, warehouse, printweigh room, maintenance shop, lab, office)	Job Title	Start Date (MM/YYYY)	End Date (MM/YYYY)	Comments

ASK THE FOLLOWING (24a-f) ABOUT EACH JOB:
a)   In this job, did you work with liquid buttermilk flavorings?

1. ___ Yes   0. ___ No

IF YES:
b) How often did you work with liquid buttermilk flavorings?

1. ___ daily
2. ___ weekly
3. ___ monthly
4. ___ < one time per month

ID _____

   c) In this job, did you work with powdered buttermilk flavorings?

                                        1. ___Yes   0. ___No

IF YES:

      d) How often did you work with powdered buttermilk flavorings

                                          1. ___ daily
                                          2. ___ weekly
                                          3. ___ monthly
                                          4. ___ < one time per month

   e) In this job, did you work with flour?

                                          1. ___Yes   0. ___No

IF YES:

      f) How often did you work with flour?

                                          1. ___ daily
                                          2. ___ weekly
                                          3. ___ monthly
                                          4. ___ < one time per month

25.   Do you use compressed air for cleaning at this facility?   1. ___Yes   0. ___No

26.   Do you wear a mask or respirator at this facility?   1. ___Yes   0. ___No
IF YES:

a)	Where do you wear the mask or respirator? *(Check all that apply)*	1. ___ production room 2. ___ lab flavoring room 3. ___ other area; Describe: _____
b)	For what tasks do you wear the mask or respirator? _____	
c)	When did you start wearing the respirator or mask?	___ / _____ (mm / yyyy)
d)	Do you wear the respirator or mask when working with buttermilk flavoring ingredients?	1. ___Yes 0. ___No 9. ___ N/A (no flavoring ingredients)
e)	Did you have a fit test for the respirator?	1. ___Yes 0. ___No 9. ___ N/A (only wore mask)

(A fit test is a test in which a technician measures how well the mask or respirator fits your face during activities such as talking and moving your head. It could involve smelling smoke, tasting something sweet or bitter, or a special machine that counts particles inside and outside the mask.)

I'm now going to ask you about all the other jobs that you have had, not at this facility.

27.   In your other jobs, not at this facility, did you work with flavoring ingredients?

                                          1. ___Yes   0. ___No

ID _____

If YES:

a)	How often did you work with flavoring ingredients:	____ daily ____ weekly ____ monthly ____ < one time per month
b)	For how many years total did you work with flavoring ingredients? ____ years	

Section IV: Tobacco Use Information

I'm now going to ask you about tobacco use.

28. Have you ever smoked cigarettes?   1. ___ Yes   0. ___ No
     (*NO if less than 20 packs of cigarettes in a*
     lifetime or less than 1 cigarette a day for 1 year.)

IF YES:

a) How old were you when you first started
    smoking regularly?   _____ Years old

b) Over the entire time that you have smoked,
    what is the average number of cigarettes
    that you smoked per day?   _____ Cigarettes/day

c) Do you still smoke cigarettes?   1. ___ Yes   0. ___ No

    IF NO:

d) How old were you when you stopped
    smoking regularly?   _____ Years old

Thank you for participating in this survey!

ACKNOWLEDGEMENTS AND AVAILABILITY OF REPORT

The Respiratory Disease Hazard Evaluation and Technical Assistance Program (RDHETAP) of NIOSH conducts field investigations of possible health hazards in the workplace. These investigations are conducted under the authority of Section 20(a)(6) of the Occupational Safety and Health (OSH) Act of 1970, 29 U.S.C. 669(a)(6), or Section 501(a)(11) of the Federal Mine Safety and Health Act of 1977, 30 U.S.C. 951(a)(11), which authorizes the Secretary of Health and Human Services, following a written request from any employers or authorized representative of employees, to determine whether any substance normally found in the place of employment has potentially toxic effects in such concentrations as used or found.

The findings and conclusions in this report are those of the authors and do not necessarily represent the views of NIOSH. Mention of any company or product does not constitute endorsement by NIOSH. In addition, citations to websites external to NIOSH do not constitute NIOSH endorsement of the sponsoring organizations or their programs or products. Furthermore, NIOSH is not responsible for the content of these websites. All Web addresses referenced in this document were accessible as of the publication date.

RDHETAP also provides, upon request, technical and consultative assistance to federal, state, and local agencies; labor; industry; and other groups or individuals to control occupational health hazards and to prevent related trauma and disease. Mention of company names or products does not constitute endorsement by NIOSH.

This report was prepared by Gregory Day, Kristin Cummings, and Greg Kullman of RDHETAP, Division of Respiratory Disease Studies. Field assistance was provided by Thomas Jefferson, Muazzam Nasrullah, Rena Saito, Jim Taylor, and Brian Tift. Data management and programming was provided by Brian Tift, Nicole Edwards, and Kathy Fedan. Desktop publishing was performed by Tia McClelland.

Copies of this report have been sent to management representatives at General Mills, Inc., HHE requestors, International Brotherhood of Teamsters, California Department of Public Health, California State OSHA, and the Federal OSHA Regional Office. This report is not copyrighted and may be freely reproduced. The report may be viewed and printed from the following internet address: http://www.cdc.gov/niosh/hhe. Copies may be purchased from the National Technical Information Service (NTIS) at 5825 Port Royal Road, Springfield, Virginia 22161.

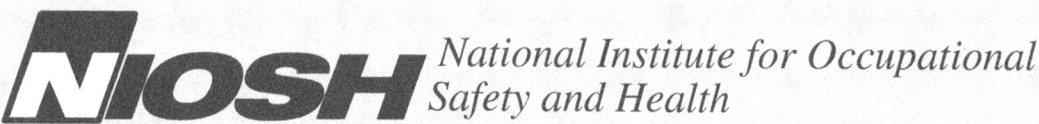

National Institute for Occupational Safety and Health

Delivering on the Nation's promise: Safety and health at work for all people through research and prevention.

To receive NIOSH documents or information about occupational safety and health topics contact NIOSH at:

1-800-35-NIOSH (1-800-356-4674)

Fax: 1-513-533-8573

E-mail: pubstaft@cdc.gov
or visit the NIOSH web site at:
http://www.cdc.gov/niosh/hhe

SAFER•HEALTHIER•PEOPLE™